Healing Salve:

30 Herbal Salves Recipes For Health And

Healing

Table of content

Introduction

Cuts. Scrapes. Burns. Let's face it, they happen. When you are active and living your life, it's only a matter of time before your body is subjected to the wear and tear of your day. You might take some precautions to keep your skin safe, but when it comes down to it, your skin is going to take the brunt of most of what you do.

To keep the damage to your skin at a minimum, you are going to have to care for it. With the use of moisturizing healing salves, you are going to give your body the moisture it needs to heal, be happy, and be healthy.

To make this even healthier, make your own healing salves and avoid the harmful chemicals that are put into the store bought salves.

Even when you are using these salves with the best intentions, when you put the salves on your body, you are also adding harmful chemicals that are doing more harm than they are good.

However, when you make your own salves, you can rest assured that there is nothing in the salves that you don't want to be in there. With the use of healing herbs and natural oils, you can apply these salves without worry that you are putting anything on your skin that you should not.

In this book, you are going to discover exactly what you need to create a variety of healing salves for all your skin care needs. From dry skin to scars to injuries, these salves are going to keep your skin happy, healthy, and strong.

Try all these recipes for yourself, and discover which works best for you. You are bound to fall in love with each of them, and your skin will thank you.

Chapter 1 – The Recipes

Super Moisture

What you will need:

8 drops myrrh oil

8 drops frankincense oil

2 cups almond oil

¼ cup beeswax

½ cup mango butter

2 tablespoons comfrey leaf

1 teaspoon rosemary leaf

1 teaspoon dried marshmallow leaf

Directions:

Grate or slice the beeswax into much smaller pieces and set aside. In a double boiler (or in a double boiler you made yourself) place the herbs with the almond oil. Turn on to low heat and simmer the herbs in the oil for 4 hours, until the oil has begun to turn a darker green color.

Once the oil has been well infused with the herbs, strain out the leaves and discard, then carefully add the mango butter and beeswax to the almond oil. Turn up the heat to medium or medium high, and allow the beeswax and almond butter to melt into the almond oil.

Once this is thoroughly melted, add in the essential oils, stirring to blend well. Remove from heat and allow the temperature to cool slightly, then transfer the mix to your individual jars.

The salve must be stored at room temperature, and can be used for up to 6 months.

Happy Hands

What you will need:

8 drops lavender oil

6 drops goldenseal oil

2 cups almond oil

¼ cup beeswax

½ cup mango butter

2 tablespoons comfrey leaf

1 teaspoon rosemary leaf

1 teaspoon dried marshmallow leaf

Directions:

Grate or slice the beeswax into much smaller pieces and set aside. In a double boiler (or in a double boiler you made yourself) place the herbs with the almond oil.

Turn on to low heat and simmer the herbs in the oil for 4 hours, until the oil has begun to turn a darker green color.

Once the oil has been well infused with the herbs, strain out the leaves and discard, then carefully add the mango butter and beeswax to the almond oil. Turn up the heat to medium or medium high, and allow the beeswax and almond butter to melt into the almond oil.

Once this is thoroughly melted, add in the essential oils, stirring to blend well. Remove from heat and allow the temperature to cool slightly, then transfer the mix to your individual jars.

The salve must be stored at room temperature, and can be used for up to 6 months.

Herbal Happiness

What you will need:

10 drops tea tree oil

10 drops myrrh oil

2 cups almond oil

¼ cup beeswax

½ cup mango butter

2 tablespoons comfrey leaf

1 teaspoon rosemary leaf

1 teaspoon dried marshmallow leaf

Directions:

Grate or slice the beeswax into much smaller pieces and set aside. In a double boiler (or in a double boiler you made yourself) place the herbs with the almond oil. Turn on to low heat and simmer the herbs in the oil for 4 hours, until the oil has begun to turn a darker green color.

Once the oil has been well infused with the herbs, strain out the leaves and discard, then carefully add the mango butter and beeswax to the almond oil.

Turn up the heat to medium or medium high, and allow the beeswax and almond butter to melt into the almond oil.

Once this is thoroughly melted, add in the essential oils, stirring to blend well. Remove from heat and allow the temperature to cool slightly, then transfer the mix to your individual jars.

The salve must be stored at room temperature, and can be used for up to 6 months.

Creamy Clean

What you will need:

10 drops basil oil

9 drops clove oil

2 cups almond oil

¼ cup beeswax

½ cup mango butter

2 tablespoons comfrey leaf

1 teaspoon rosemary leaf

1 teaspoon dried marshmallow leaf

Directions:

Grate or slice the beeswax into much smaller pieces and set aside. In a double boiler (or in a double boiler you made yourself) place the herbs with the almond oil. Turn on to low heat and simmer the herbs in the oil for 4 hours, until the oil has begun to turn a darker green color.

Once the oil has been well infused with the herbs, strain out the leaves and discard, then carefully add the mango butter and beeswax to the almond oil. Turn up the heat to medium or medium high, and allow the beeswax and almond butter to melt into the almond oil.

Once this is thoroughly melted, add in the essential oils, stirring to blend well. Remove from heat and allow the temperature to cool slightly, then transfer the mix to your individual jars.

The salve must be stored at room temperature, and can be used for up to 6 months.

Go Moisture

What you will need:

10 drops vanilla oil

10 drops geranium oil

2 cups almond oil

¼ cup beeswax

½ cup mango butter

2 tablespoons comfrey leaf

1 teaspoon rosemary leaf

1 teaspoon dried marshmallow leaf

Directions:

Grate or slice the beeswax into much smaller pieces and set aside. In a double boiler (or in a double boiler you made yourself) place the herbs with the almond oil. Turn on to low heat and simmer the herbs in the oil for 4 hours, until the oil has begun to turn a darker green color.

Once the oil has been well infused with the herbs, strain out the leaves and discard, then carefully add the mango butter and beeswax to the almond oil. Turn up the heat to medium or medium high, and allow the beeswax and almond butter to melt into the almond oil.

Once this is thoroughly melted, add in the essential oils, stirring to blend well. Remove from heat and allow the temperature to cool slightly, then transfer the mix to your individual jars.

The salve must be stored at room temperature, and can be used for up to 6 months.

Smooth as Silk

What you will need:

10 drops lemon oil

10 drops lemongrass oil

2 cups almond oil

¼ cup beeswax

½ cup mango butter

2 tablespoons comfrey leaf

1 teaspoon rosemary leaf

1 teaspoon dried marshmallow leaf

Directions:

Grate or slice the beeswax into much smaller pieces and set aside. In a double boiler (or in a double boiler you made yourself) place the herbs with the almond oil. Turn on to low heat and simmer the herbs in the oil for 4 hours, until the oil has begun to turn a darker green color.

Once the oil has been well infused with the herbs, strain out the leaves and discard, then carefully add the mango butter and beeswax to the almond oil. Turn up the heat to medium or medium high, and allow the beeswax and almond butter to melt into the almond oil.

Once this is thoroughly melted, add in the essential oils, stirring to blend well. Remove from heat and allow the temperature to cool slightly, then transfer the mix to your individual jars.

The salve must be stored at room temperature, and can be used for up to 6 months.

Satin Skin

What you will need:

10 drops lemongrass oil

11 drops wheatgrass oil

2 cups almond oil

¼ cup beeswax

½ cup mango butter

2 tablespoons comfrey leaf

1 teaspoon rosemary leaf

1 teaspoon dried marshmallow leaf

Directions:

Grate or slice the beeswax into much smaller pieces and set aside. In a double boiler (or in a double boiler you made yourself) place the herbs with the almond oil. Turn on to low heat and simmer the herbs in the oil for 4 hours, until the oil has begun to turn a darker green color.

Once the oil has been well infused with the herbs, strain out the leaves and discard, then carefully add the mango butter and beeswax to the almond oil. Turn up the heat to medium or medium high, and allow the beeswax and almond butter to melt into the almond oil.

Once this is thoroughly melted, add in the essential oils, stirring to blend well. Remove from heat and allow the temperature to cool slightly, then transfer the mix to your individual jars.

The salve must be stored at room temperature, and can be used for up to 6 months.

Scar Banisher

What you will need:

10 drops myrrh oil

10 drops grapefruit oil

2 cups almond oil

¼ cup beeswax

½ cup mango butter

2 tablespoons comfrey leaf

1 teaspoon rosemary leaf

1 teaspoon dried marshmallow leaf

Directions:

Grate or slice the beeswax into much smaller pieces and set aside. In a double boiler (or in a double boiler you made yourself) place the herbs with the almond oil. Turn on to low heat and simmer the herbs in the oil for 4 hours, until the oil has begun to turn a darker green color.

Once the oil has been well infused with the herbs, strain out the leaves and discard, then carefully add the mango butter and beeswax to the almond oil. Turn up the heat to medium or medium high, and allow the beeswax and almond butter to melt into the almond oil.

Once this is thoroughly melted, add in the essential oils, stirring to blend well. Remove from heat and allow the temperature to cool slightly, then transfer the mix to your individual jars.

The salve must be stored at room temperature, and can be used for up to 6 months.

Hurt Healer

What you will need:

19 drops orange oil

11 drops blood orange oil

2 cups almond oil

¼ cup beeswax

½ cup mango butter

2 tablespoons comfrey leaf

1 teaspoon rosemary leaf

1 teaspoon dried marshmallow leaf

Directions:

Grate or slice the beeswax into much smaller pieces and set aside. In a double boiler (or in a double boiler you made yourself) place the herbs with the almond oil. Turn on to low heat and simmer the herbs in the oil for 4 hours, until the oil has begun to turn a darker green color.

Once the oil has been well infused with the herbs, strain out the leaves and discard, then carefully add the mango butter and beeswax to the almond oil. Turn up the heat to medium or medium high, and allow the beeswax and almond butter to melt into the almond oil.

Once this is thoroughly melted, add in the essential oils, stirring to blend well. Remove from heat and allow the temperature to cool slightly, then transfer the mix to your individual jars.

The salve must be stored at room temperature, and can be used for up to 6 months.

Peppermint Power

What you will need:

10 drops peppermint oil

10 drops mint oil

2 cups almond oil

¼ cup beeswax

½ cup mango butter

2 tablespoons comfrey leaf

1 teaspoon rosemary leaf

1 teaspoon dried marshmallow leaf

Directions:

Grate or slice the beeswax into much smaller pieces and set aside. In a double boiler (or in a double boiler you made yourself) place the herbs with the almond oil. Turn on to low heat and simmer the herbs in the oil for 4 hours, until the oil has begun to turn a darker green color.

Once the oil has been well infused with the herbs, strain out the leaves and discard, then carefully add the mango butter and beeswax to the almond oil. Turn up the heat to medium or medium high, and allow the beeswax and almond butter to melt into the almond oil.

Once this is thoroughly melted, add in the essential oils, stirring to blend well. Remove from heat and allow the temperature to cool slightly, then transfer the mix to your individual jars.

The salve must be stored at room temperature, and can be used for up to 6 months.

Germm Fighter

What you will need:

10 drops tea tree oil

10 drops orange oil

2 cups almond oil

¼ cup beeswax

½ cup mango butter

2 tablespoons comfrey leaf

1 teaspoon rosemary leaf

1 teaspoon dried marshmallow leaf

Directions:

Grate or slice the beeswax into much smaller pieces and set aside. In a double boiler (or in a double boiler you made yourself) place the herbs with the almond oil. Turn on to low heat and simmer the herbs in the oil for 4 hours, until the oil has begun to turn a darker green color.

Once the oil has been well infused with the herbs, strain out the leaves and discard, then carefully add the mango butter and beeswax to the almond oil. Turn up the heat to medium or medium high, and allow the beeswax and almond butter to melt into the almond oil.

Once this is thoroughly melted, add in the essential oils, stirring to blend well. Remove from heat and allow the temperature to cool slightly, then transfer the mix to your individual jars.

The salve must be stored at room temperature, and can be used for up to 6 months.

Callous Clash

What you will need:

10 drops myrrh oil

11 drops cinnamon oil

2 cups almond oil

¼ cup beeswax

½ cup mango butter

2 tablespoons comfrey leaf

1 teaspoon rosemary leaf

1 teaspoon dried marshmallow leaf

Directions:

Grate or slice the beeswax into much smaller pieces and set aside. In a double boiler (or in a double boiler you made yourself) place the herbs with the almond oil. Turn on to low heat and simmer the herbs in the oil for 4 hours, until the oil has begun to turn a darker green color.

Once the oil has been well infused with the herbs, strain out the leaves and discard, then carefully add the mango butter and beeswax to the almond oil. Turn up the heat to medium or medium high, and allow the beeswax and almond butter to melt into the almond oil.

Once this is thoroughly melted, add in the essential oils, stirring to blend well. Remove from heat and allow the temperature to cool slightly, then transfer the mix to your individual jars.

The salve must be stored at room temperature, and can be used for up to 6 months.

Dessert Oasis

What you will need:

19 drops lemon oil

11 drops orange oil

2 cups almond oil

¼ cup beeswax

½ cup mango butter

2 tablespoons comfrey leaf

1 teaspoon rosemary leaf

1 teaspoon dried marshmallow leaf

Directions:

Grate or slice the beeswax into much smaller pieces and set aside. In a double boiler (or in a double boiler you made yourself) place the herbs with the almond oil. Turn on to low heat and simmer the herbs in the oil for 4 hours, until the oil has begun to turn a darker green color.

Once the oil has been well infused with the herbs, strain out the leaves and discard, then carefully add the mango butter and beeswax to the almond oil. Turn up the heat to medium or medium high, and allow the beeswax and almond butter to melt into the almond oil.

Once this is thoroughly melted, add in the essential oils, stirring to blend well. Remove from heat and allow the temperature to cool slightly, then transfer the mix to your individual jars.

The salve must be stored at room temperature, and can be used for up to 6 months.

Knuckle Smoother

What you will need:

11 drops peppermint oil

11 drops grapefruit oil

2 cups almond oil

¼ cup beeswax

½ cup mango butter

2 tablespoons comfrey leaf

1 teaspoon rosemary leaf

1 teaspoon dried marshmallow leaf

Directions:

Grate or slice the beeswax into much smaller pieces and set aside. In a double boiler (or in a double boiler you made yourself) place the herbs with the almond oil. Turn on to low heat and simmer the herbs in the oil for 4 hours, until the oil has begun to turn a darker green color.

Once the oil has been well infused with the herbs, strain out the leaves and discard, then carefully add the mango butter and beeswax to the almond oil. Turn up the heat to medium or medium high, and allow the beeswax and almond butter to melt into the almond oil.

Once this is thoroughly melted, add in the essential oils, stirring to blend well. Remove from heat and allow the temperature to cool slightly, then transfer the mix to your individual jars.

The salve must be stored at room temperature, and can be used for up to 6 months.

The Giggler

What you will need:

10 drops grapefruit

12 drops blood orange oil

2 cups almond oil

¼ cup beeswax

½ cup mango butter

2 tablespoons comfrey leaf

1 teaspoon rosemary leaf

1 teaspoon dried marshmallow leaf

Directions:

Grate or slice the beeswax into much smaller pieces and set aside. In a double boiler (or in a double boiler you made yourself) place the herbs with the almond oil. Turn on to low heat and simmer the herbs in the oil for 4 hours, until the oil has begun to turn a darker green color.

Once the oil has been well infused with the herbs, strain out the leaves and discard, then carefully add the mango butter and beeswax to the almond oil. Turn up the heat to medium or medium high, and allow the beeswax and almond butter to melt into the almond oil.

Once this is thoroughly melted, add in the essential oils, stirring to blend well. Remove from heat and allow the temperature to cool slightly, then transfer the mix to your individual jars.

The salve must be stored at room temperature, and can be used for up to 6 months.

Beautiful

What you will need:

10 drops rose oil

11 drops lavender oil

2 cups almond oil

¼ cup beeswax

½ cup mango butter

2 tablespoons comfrey leaf

1 teaspoon rosemary leaf

1 teaspoon dried marshmallow leaf

Directions:

Grate or slice the beeswax into much smaller pieces and set aside. In a double boiler (or in a double boiler you made yourself) place the herbs with the almond oil. Turn on to low heat and simmer the herbs in the oil for 4 hours, until the oil has begun to turn a darker green color.

Once the oil has been well infused with the herbs, strain out the leaves and discard, then carefully add the mango butter and beeswax to the almond oil. Turn up the heat to medium or medium high, and allow the beeswax and almond butter to melt into the almond oil.

Once this is thoroughly melted, add in the essential oils, stirring to blend well. Remove from heat and allow the temperature to cool slightly, then transfer the mix to your individual jars.

The salve must be stored at room temperature, and can be used for up to 6 months.

Princess Hands

What you will need:

12 drops geranium oil

12 drops vanilla oil

2 cups almond oil

¼ cup beeswax

½ cup mango butter

2 tablespoons comfrey leaf

1 teaspoon rosemary leaf

1 teaspoon dried marshmallow leaf

Directions:

Grate or slice the beeswax into much smaller pieces and set aside. In a double boiler (or in a double boiler you made yourself) place the herbs with the almond oil. Turn on to low heat and simmer the herbs in the oil for 4 hours, until the oil has begun to turn a darker green color.

Once the oil has been well infused with the herbs, strain out the leaves and discard, then carefully add the mango butter and beeswax to the almond oil. Turn up the heat to medium or medium high, and allow the beeswax and almond butter to melt into the almond oil.

Once this is thoroughly melted, add in the essential oils, stirring to blend well. Remove from heat and allow the temperature to cool slightly, then transfer the mix to your individual jars.

The salve must be stored at room temperature, and can be used for up to 6 months.

It's in the Knees

What you will need:

10 drops myrrh oil

11 drops spearmint oil

2 cups almond oil

¼ cup beeswax

½ cup mango butter

2 tablespoons comfrey leaf

1 teaspoon rosemary leaf

1 teaspoon dried marshmallow leaf

Directions:

Grate or slice the beeswax into much smaller pieces and set aside. In a double boiler (or in a double boiler you made yourself) place the herbs with the almond oil. Turn on to low heat and simmer the herbs in the oil for 4 hours, until the oil has begun to turn a darker green color.

Once the oil has been well infused with the herbs, strain out the leaves and discard, then carefully add the mango butter and beeswax to the almond oil. Turn up the heat to medium or medium high, and allow the beeswax and almond butter to melt into the almond oil.

Once this is thoroughly melted, add in the essential oils, stirring to blend well. Remove from heat and allow the temperature to cool slightly, then transfer the mix to your individual jars.

The salve must be stored at room temperature, and can be used for up to 6 months.

No More Scabs

What you will need:

12 drops lemon oil

12 drops chamomile oil

2 cups almond oil

¼ cup beeswax

½ cup mango butter

2 tablespoons comfrey leaf

1 teaspoon rosemary leaf

1 teaspoon dried marshmallow leaf

Directions:

Grate or slice the beeswax into much smaller pieces and set aside. In a double boiler (or in a double boiler you made yourself) place the herbs with the almond oil. Turn on to low heat and simmer the herbs in the oil for 4 hours, until the oil has begun to turn a darker green color.

Once the oil has been well infused with the herbs, strain out the leaves and discard, then carefully add the mango butter and beeswax to the almond oil. Turn up the heat to medium or medium high, and allow the beeswax and almond butter to melt into the almond oil.

Once this is thoroughly melted, add in the essential oils, stirring to blend well. Remove from heat and allow the temperature to cool slightly, then transfer the mix to your individual jars.

The salve must be stored at room temperature, and can be used for up to 6 months.

Sunburn Fixer

What you will need:

19 drops lemon oil

12 drops vetiver oil

2 cups almond oil

¼ cup beeswax

½ cup mango butter

2 tablespoons comfrey leaf

1 teaspoon rosemary leaf

1 teaspoon dried marshmallow leaf

Directions:

Grate or slice the beeswax into much smaller pieces and set aside. In a double boiler (or in a double boiler you made yourself) place the herbs with the almond oil. Turn on to low heat and simmer the herbs in the oil for 4 hours, until the oil has begun to turn a darker green color.

Once the oil has been well infused with the herbs, strain out the leaves and discard, then carefully add the mango butter and beeswax to the almond oil. Turn up the heat to medium or medium high, and allow the beeswax and almond butter to melt into the almond oil.

Once this is thoroughly melted, add in the essential oils, stirring to blend well. Remove from heat and allow the temperature to cool slightly, then transfer the mix to your individual jars.

The salve must be stored at room temperature, and can be used for up to 6 months.

Summer's Sunshine

What you will need:

10 drops ylang ylang

12 drops vanilla oil

2 cups almond oil

¼ cup beeswax

½ cup mango butter

2 tablespoons comfrey leaf

1 teaspoon rosemary leaf

1 teaspoon dried marshmallow leaf

Directions:

Grate or slice the beeswax into much smaller pieces and set aside. In a double boiler (or in a double boiler you made yourself) place the herbs with the almond oil. Turn on to low heat and simmer the herbs in the oil for 4 hours, until the oil has begun to turn a darker green color.

Once the oil has been well infused with the herbs, strain out the leaves and discard, then carefully add the mango butter and beeswax to the almond oil. Turn up the heat to medium or medium high, and allow the beeswax and almond butter to melt into the almond oil.

Once this is thoroughly melted, add in the essential oils, stirring to blend well. Remove from heat and allow the temperature to cool slightly, then transfer the mix to your individual jars.

The salve must be stored at room temperature, and can be used for up to 6 months.

Shake My Hand

What you will need:

10 drops cinnamon oil

12 drops ginger oil

2 cups almond oil

¼ cup beeswax

½ cup mango butter

2 tablespoons comfrey leaf

1 teaspoon rosemary leaf

1 teaspoon dried marshmallow leaf

Directions:

Grate or slice the beeswax into much smaller pieces and set aside. In a double boiler (or in a double boiler you made yourself) place the herbs with the almond oil. Turn on to low heat and simmer the herbs in the oil for 4 hours, until the oil has begun to turn a darker green color.

Once the oil has been well infused with the herbs, strain out the leaves and discard, then carefully add the mango butter and beeswax to the almond oil. Turn up the heat to medium or medium high, and allow the beeswax and almond butter to melt into the almond oil.

Once this is thoroughly melted, add in the essential oils, stirring to blend well. Remove from heat and allow the temperature to cool slightly, then transfer the mix to your individual jars.

The salve must be stored at room temperature, and can be used for up to 6 months.

All Over Moisture

What you will need:

12 drops eucalyptus oil

10 drops spearmint oil

2 cups almond oil

¼ cup beeswax

½ cup mango butter

2 tablespoons comfrey leaf

1 teaspoon rosemary leaf

1 teaspoon dried marshmallow leaf

Directions:

Grate or slice the beeswax into much smaller pieces and set aside. In a double boiler (or in a double boiler you made yourself) place the herbs with the almond oil. Turn on to low heat and simmer the herbs in the oil for 4 hours, until the oil has begun to turn a darker green color.

Once the oil has been well infused with the herbs, strain out the leaves and discard, then carefully add the mango butter and beeswax to the almond oil. Turn up the heat to medium or medium high, and allow the beeswax and almond butter to melt into the almond oil.

Once this is thoroughly melted, add in the essential oils, stirring to blend well. Remove from heat and allow the temperature to cool slightly, then transfer the mix to your individual jars.

The salve must be stored at room temperature, and can be used for up to 6 months.

Million Dollar Moisture

What you will need:

12 drops cedar oil

11 drops sandalwood oil

2 cups almond oil

¼ cup beeswax

½ cup mango butter

2 tablespoons comfrey leaf

1 teaspoon rosemary leaf

1 teaspoon dried marshmallow leaf

Directions:

Grate or slice the beeswax into much smaller pieces and set aside. In a double boiler (or in a double boiler you made yourself) place the herbs with the almond oil. Turn on to low heat and simmer the herbs in the oil for 4 hours, until the oil has begun to turn a darker green color.

Once the oil has been well infused with the herbs, strain out the leaves and discard, then carefully add the mango butter and beeswax to the almond oil. Turn up the heat to medium or medium high, and allow the beeswax and almond butter to melt into the almond oil.

Once this is thoroughly melted, add in the essential oils, stirring to blend well. Remove from heat and allow the temperature to cool slightly, then transfer the mix to your individual jars.

The salve must be stored at room temperature, and can be used for up to 6 months.

Moisture in the Mix

What you will need:

12 drops myrrh oil

10 drops vetiver oil

2 cups almond oil

¼ cup beeswax

½ cup mango butter

2 tablespoons comfrey leaf

1 teaspoon rosemary leaf

1 teaspoon dried marshmallow leaf

Directions:

Grate or slice the beeswax into much smaller pieces and set aside. In a double boiler (or in a double boiler you made yourself) place the herbs with the almond oil. Turn on to low heat and simmer the herbs in the oil for 4 hours, until the oil has begun to turn a darker green color.

Once the oil has been well infused with the herbs, strain out the leaves and discard, then carefully add the mango butter and beeswax to the almond oil. Turn up the heat to medium or medium high, and allow the beeswax and almond butter to melt into the almond oil.

Once this is thoroughly melted, add in the essential oils, stirring to blend well. Remove from heat and allow the temperature to cool slightly, then transfer the mix to your individual jars.

The salve must be stored at room temperature, and can be used for up to 6 months.

Savannah Sunshine

What you will need:

10 drops geranium oil

14 drops sandalwood oil

2 cups almond oil

¼ cup beeswax

½ cup mango butter

2 tablespoons comfrey leaf

1 teaspoon rosemary leaf

1 teaspoon dried marshmallow leaf

Directions:

Grate or slice the beeswax into much smaller pieces and set aside. In a double boiler (or in a double boiler you made yourself) place the herbs with the almond oil. Turn on to low heat and simmer the herbs in the oil for 4 hours, until the oil has begun to turn a darker green color.

Once the oil has been well infused with the herbs, strain out the leaves and discard, then carefully add the mango butter and beeswax to the almond oil. Turn up the heat to medium or medium high, and allow the beeswax and almond butter to melt into the almond oil.

Once this is thoroughly melted, add in the essential oils, stirring to blend well. Remove from heat and allow the temperature to cool slightly, then transfer the mix to your individual jars.

The salve must be stored at room temperature, and can be used for up to 6 months.

Dessert Rain

What you will need:

10 drops cinnamon oil

12 drops ylang ylang oil

2 cups almond oil

¼ cup beeswax

½ cup mango butter

2 tablespoons comfrey leaf

1 teaspoon rosemary leaf

1 teaspoon dried marshmallow leaf

Directions:

Grate or slice the beeswax into much smaller pieces and set aside. In a double boiler (or in a double boiler you made yourself) place the herbs with the almond oil. Turn on to low heat and simmer the herbs in the oil for 4 hours, until the oil has begun to turn a darker green color.

Once the oil has been well infused with the herbs, strain out the leaves and discard, then carefully add the mango butter and beeswax to the almond oil. Turn up the heat to medium or medium high, and allow the beeswax and almond butter to melt into the almond oil.

Once this is thoroughly melted, add in the essential oils, stirring to blend well. Remove from heat and allow the temperature to cool slightly, then transfer the mix to your individual jars.

The salve must be stored at room temperature, and can be used for up to 6 months.

Splash Salve

What you will need:

10 drops balsam fir oil

8 drops chamomile oil

2 cups almond oil

¼ cup beeswax

½ cup mango butter

2 tablespoons comfrey leaf

1 teaspoon rosemary leaf

1 teaspoon dried marshmallow leaf

Directions:

Grate or slice the beeswax into much smaller pieces and set aside. In a double boiler (or in a double boiler you made yourself) place the herbs with the almond oil. Turn on to low heat and simmer the herbs in the oil for 4 hours, until the oil has begun to turn a darker green color.

Once the oil has been well infused with the herbs, strain out the leaves and discard, then carefully add the mango butter and beeswax to the almond oil. Turn up the heat to medium or medium high, and allow the beeswax and almond butter to melt into the almond oil.

Once this is thoroughly melted, add in the essential oils, stirring to blend well. Remove from heat and allow the temperature to cool slightly, then transfer the mix to your individual jars.

The salve must be stored at room temperature, and can be used for up to 6 months.

Bliss

What you will need:

12 drops sunflower oil

12 drops peppermint oil

2 cups almond oil

¼ cup beeswax

½ cup mango butter

2 tablespoons comfrey leaf

1 teaspoon rosemary leaf

1 teaspoon dried marshmallow leaf

Directions:

Grate or slice the beeswax into much smaller pieces and set aside. In a double boiler (or in a double boiler you made yourself) place the herbs with the almond oil. Turn on to low heat and simmer the herbs in the oil for 4 hours, until the oil has begun to turn a darker green color.

Once the oil has been well infused with the herbs, strain out the leaves and discard, then carefully add the mango butter and beeswax to the almond oil. Turn up the heat to medium or medium high, and allow the beeswax and almond butter to melt into the almond oil.

Once this is thoroughly melted, add in the essential oils, stirring to blend well. Remove from heat and allow the temperature to cool slightly, then transfer the mix to your individual jars.

The salve must be stored at room temperature, and can be used for up to 6 months.

Juicy Drops

What you will need:

10 drops orange oil

10 drops bergamot oil

2 cups almond oil

¼ cup beeswax

½ cup mango butter

2 tablespoons comfrey leaf

1 teaspoon rosemary leaf

1 teaspoon dried marshmallow leaf

Directions:

Grate or slice the beeswax into much smaller pieces and set aside. In a double boiler (or in a double boiler you made yourself) place the herbs with the almond oil. Turn on to low heat and simmer the herbs in the oil for 4 hours, until the oil has begun to turn a darker green color.

Once the oil has been well infused with the herbs, strain out the leaves and discard, then carefully add the mango butter and beeswax to the almond oil. Turn up the heat to medium or medium high, and allow the beeswax and almond butter to melt into the almond oil.

Once this is thoroughly melted, add in the essential oils, stirring to blend well. Remove from heat and allow the temperature to cool slightly, then transfer the mix to your individual jars.

The salve must be stored at room temperature, and can be used for up to 6 months.

Conclusion

There you have it, everything you need to know to get started making your own homemade healing salves, and what you need for a variety of different conditions. When you are making your own salves, you have everything you need to give your body moisture and healing properties, without having to turn to harmful chemicals.

I hope this book inspires you to make the best healing salves you can possibly make, and that you enjoy using these healing salves in your medicine cabinet and on your body.

There are a variety of ways you can better your health when you make your own remedies, and this book is the very tool you need to make that happen.

Experience a wealth of new health with these recipes, and achieve the perfect glowing skin!

Made in United States
Troutdale, OR
08/23/2024